The Ultimate Lean & Green Snack And Dessert Cookbook

Delicious Lean & Green Snacks And Desserts For Weight Loss

Jesse Cohen

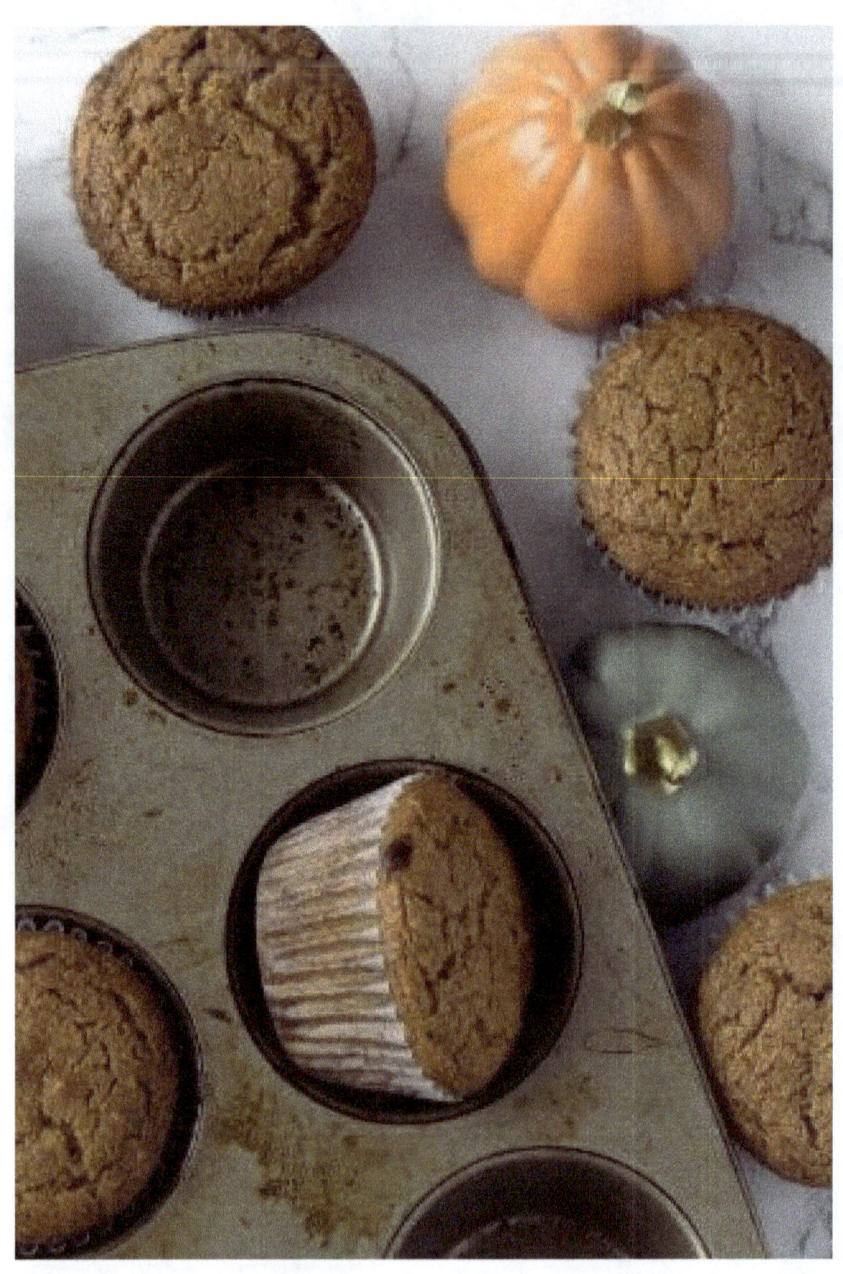

© Copyright 2020 - All rights reserved.

The content contained within this book may not be reproduced, duplicated or transmitted without direct written permission from the author or the publisher.

Under no circumstances will any blame or legal responsibility be held against the publisher, or author, for any damages, reparation, or monetary loss due to the information contained within this book. Either directly or indirectly.

Legal Notice:

This book is copyright protected. This book is only for personal use. You cannot amend, distribute, sell, use, quote or paraphrase any part, or the content within this book, without the consent of the author or publisher.

Disclaimer Notice:

Please note the information contained within this document is for educational and entertainment purposes only. All effort has been executed to present accurate, up to date, and reliable, complete information. No warranties of any kind are declared or implied. Readers acknowledge that the author is not engaging in the rendering of legal, financial, medical or professional advice. The content within this book has been derived from various sources. Please consult a licensed professional before attempting any techniques outlined in this book.

By reading this document, the reader agrees that under no circumstances is the author responsible for any losses, direct or indirect, which are incurred as a result of the use of information contained within this document, including, but not limited to, — errors, omissions, or inaccuracies.

Table of contents

Mozzarella Sticks 7

Sausage and Cheese Dip 10

Stuffed Avocado 12

Tasty Onion and Cauliflower Dip 14

Avocado Taco Boats 16

Pesto Crackers 19

Chicken and Mushrooms 21

Marinated Eggs 24

Lamb Stuffed Avocado 27

Chili Mango and Watermelon Salsa 29

Pumpkin Muffins 31

Chicken Enchilada Bake 34

Greek Tuna Salad Bites 37

Veggie Fritters 39

Olives and Cheese Stuffed Tomatoes 42

Cucumber Sandwich Bites 44

White Bean Dip 46

Eggplant Dip 48

Tomato Salsa 50

Feta Artichoke Dip 52

Bulgur Lamb Meatballs	54
Cucumber Bites	56
Hummus with Ground Lamb	58
Wrapped Plums	60
Cucumber Rolls	62
Creamy Spinach and Shallots Dip	64
Avocado Dip	66
Goat Cheese and Chives Spread	68
Chia Pudding	70
Avocado Pudding	72
Smooth Peanut Butter Cream	74
Raspberry Ice Cream	76
Chocolate Frosty	78
Cranberry Muffins	80
Bounty Bars	83
Delicious Brownie Bites	86
Chocolate Popsicle	88
Pumpkin Balls	90
Blueberry Muffins	92
Vanilla Avocado Popsicles	94
Green Pea Guacamole	96
Crispy Rye Bread Snacks with Guacamole and Anchovies	98

Chocolate Almond Butter Brownie 100

Peanut Butter Fudge 102

Almond Butter Fudge 104

Lean Granola 106

Mozzarella Sticks

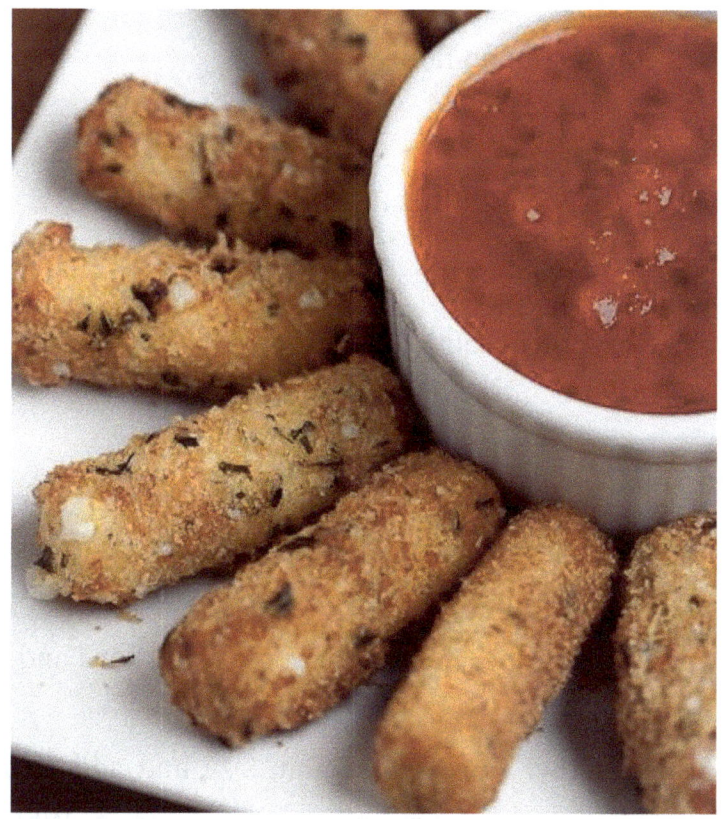

Preparation Time: 8 minutes

Cooking Time: 2 minutes

Servings: 2

Ingredients:

- 1 large whole egg

- 3 sticks of mozzarella cheese in half (frozen overnight)
- 2 tablespoon of grated parmesan cheese
- 1/2 cup of almond flour
- 1/4 cup of coconut oil
- 2 1/2 teaspoons of Italian seasoning blend
- 1 tablespoon of chopped parsley
- 1/2 teaspoon of salt

Directions:

1. Heat the coconut oil in a medium sized cast-iron skillet over low-medium heat.
2. In the meantime, crack the egg in a small bowl and beat it well.
3. Take another bowl of medium size and add parmesan cheese, almond flour, and seasonings to it. Whisk the ingredients together until a smooth mixture is available.
4. Take the overnight frozen mozzarella stick and dip it in the beaten egg, then coat it well with the dry mixture. Do the same with all the remaining cheese sticks.
5. Place all the coated sticks in the preheated skillet and cook them for 2 minutes or until they start having a golden brown look on all sides.

6. Remove from the skillet once cooked properly and place over a towel so that any extra oil gets absorbed.
7. Sprinkle parsley over the sticks if you desire and serve with keto marinara sauce.

Nutrition:

- Calories: 430 g
- Fat: 39 g
- Carbohydrates: 10 g
- Protein: 20 g

Sausage and Cheese Dip

Preparation Time: 10 minutes

Cooking Time: 130 minutes

Servings: 28

Ingredients:

- 8 ounces cream cheese
- A pinch of salt and black pepper
- 16 ounces of sour cream
- 8 ounces of pepper jack cheese; chopped
- 15 ounces of canned tomatoes mixed with habaneros
- 1-pound of Italian sausage; ground
- ¼ cup of green onions; chopped

Directions:

1. Heat up a pan over medium heat, add sausage, stir and cook until it browns.
2. Add tomatoes mix, stir and cook for 4 minutes more.
3. Add a pinch of salt, black pepper, and the green onions, stir and cook for 4 minutes.

4. Spread pepper jack cheese on the bottom of your slow cooker.
5. Add cream cheese, sausage mix, and soured cream, cover and cook on High for 2 hours.
6. Uncover your slow cooker, stir dip, transfer to a bowl, and serve.
7. Enjoy!

Nutrition:

- Calories: 132
- Protein: 6.79 g
- Fat: 9.58 g
- Carbohydrates: 6.22 g
- Sodium: 362 mg

Stuffed Avocado

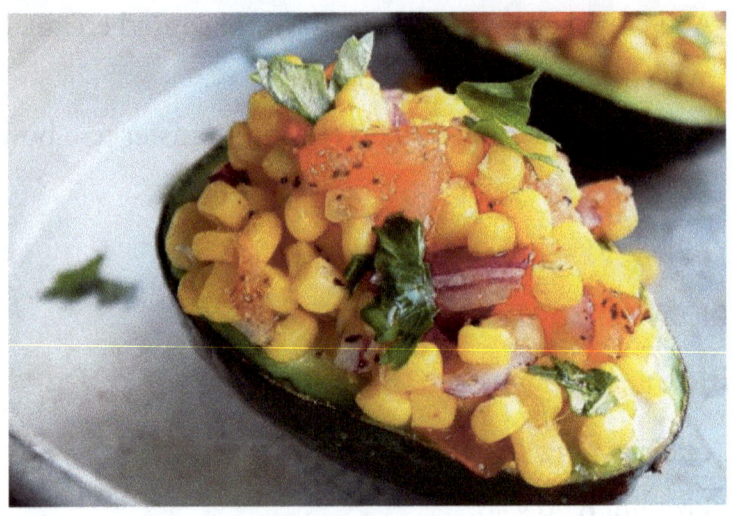

Preparation Time: 10 minutes

Cooking Time: 0 minute

Servings: 2

Ingredients:

- 1 avocado; halved and pitted
- 10 ounces of canned tuna; drained
- 2 tablespoons of sun-dried tomatoes; chopped
- 1 and ½ tablespoon of basil pesto
- 2 tablespoons of black olives; pitted and chopped

- Salt and black pepper to the taste
- 2 teaspoons of pine nuts; toasted and chopped
- 1 tablespoon of basil; chopped

Directions:

1. In a bowl, mix the tuna with the sun-dried tomatoes and the rest of the ingredients except the avocado and stir.
2. Stuff the avocado halves with the tuna mix and serve as an appetizer.

Nutrition:

- Calories: 233
- Fat: 9 g
- Fiber: 3.5 g
- Carbs: 11.4 g
- Protein: 5.6 g

Tasty Onion and Cauliflower Dip

Preparation Time: 20 minutes

Cooking Time: 30 minutes

Servings: 24

Ingredients:

- 1 ½ cups of chicken stock
- 1 cauliflower head; florets separated
- ¼ cup of mayonnaise
- ½ cup of yellow onion; chopped
- ¾ cup of cream cheese
- ½ teaspoon of chili powder
- ½ teaspoon of cumin; ground
- ½ teaspoon of garlic powder
- Salt and black pepper to the taste

Directions:

1. Put the stock in a pot, add cauliflower and onion, heat up over medium heat, and cook for 30 minutes.

2. Add chili powder, salt, pepper, cumin, garlic powder, and stir.
3. Also, add cheese and stir a touch until it melts.
4. Blend using an immersion blender and blend with the mayo.
5. Transfer to a bowl and keep in the fridge for 2 hours before you serve it.
6. Enjoy!

Nutrition:

- Calories: 40
- Protein: 1.23 g
- Fat: 3.31 g
- Carbohydrates: 1.66 g
- Sodium: 72 mg

Avocado Taco Boats

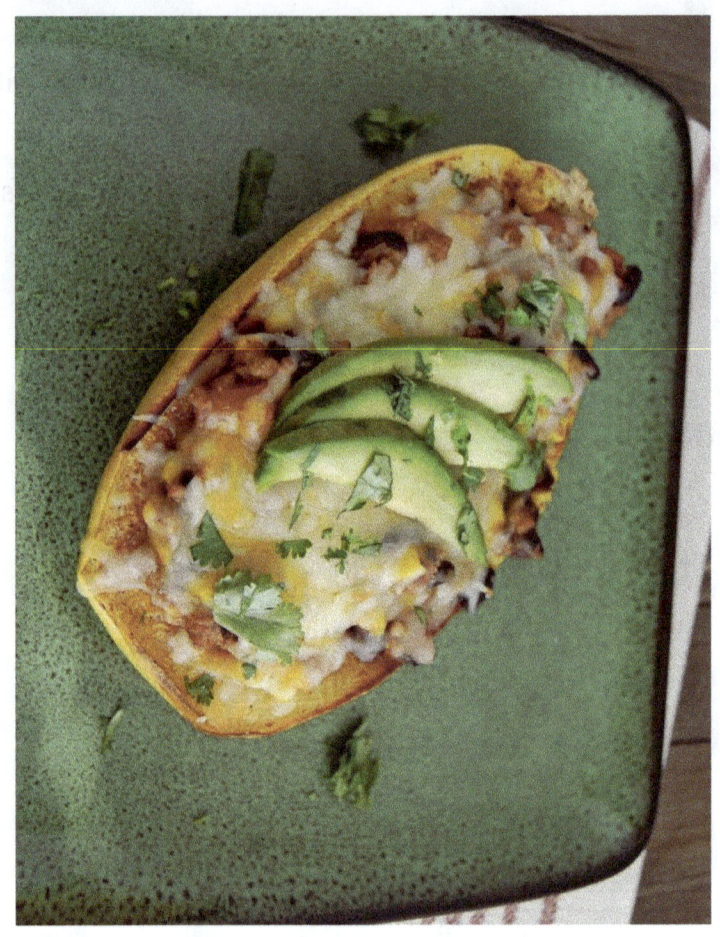

Preparation Time: 5 minutes

Cooking Time: 20 minutes

Servings: 4

Ingredients:

- 4 grape tomatoes
- 2 large avocados
- 1 lb. of ground beef
- 4 tablespoon of taco seasoning
- 3/4 cup of shredded sharp cheddar cheese
- 4 slices of pickled jalapeño
- 1/4 cup of salsa
- 3 shredded romaine leaves
- 1/4 cup of sour cream
- 2/3 cup of water

Directions:

1. Take a skillet of huge size, grease it with oil, and warmth it over medium-high heat. Cook the bottom beef in it for 10-15 minutes or until it has a brownish look.
2. Once the meat browns, drain the grease from the skillet and add the water and the taco seasoning.
3. Reduce the heat once the taco seasoning gets mixed well and simmer for 8-10 minutes.
4. Take both avocados and cut in halves using a sharp knife.

5. Take each avocado shell and fill it with ¼ of the shredded romaine leaves.
6. Fill each shell with ¼ of the cooked ground beef.
7. Do the topping with soured cream, cheese, jalapeno, salsa, and tomato before you serve the delicious avocado taco.

Nutrition:

- Calories: 430
- Fat: 35 g
- Carbohydrates: 5 g
- Protein: 32 g

Pesto Crackers

Preparation Time: 10 minutes

Cooking Time: 17 minutes

Servings: 6

Ingredients:

- ½ teaspoon of baking powder
- Salt and black pepper to the taste
- 1 and ¼ cups of almond flour
- ¼ teaspoon of basil; dried
- 1 garlic clove; minced
- 2 tablespoons of basil pesto
- A pinch of cayenne pepper
- 3 tablespoons of ghee

Directions:

1. In a bowl, mix salt, pepper, baking powder, and almond flour.
2. Add garlic, cayenne, and basil and stir.
3. Add pesto and whisk.

4. Also, add ghee and blend your dough with your finger.
5. Spread this dough on a lined baking sheet, then put in the oven at 325° F and bake for 17 minutes.
6. Set aside to cool, then cut your crackers and serve them as a snack.
7. Enjoy!

Nutrition:

- Calories: 9
- Protein: 0.41 g
- Fat: 0.14 g
- Carbohydrates: 1.86 g
- Sodium: 2 mg

Chicken and Mushrooms

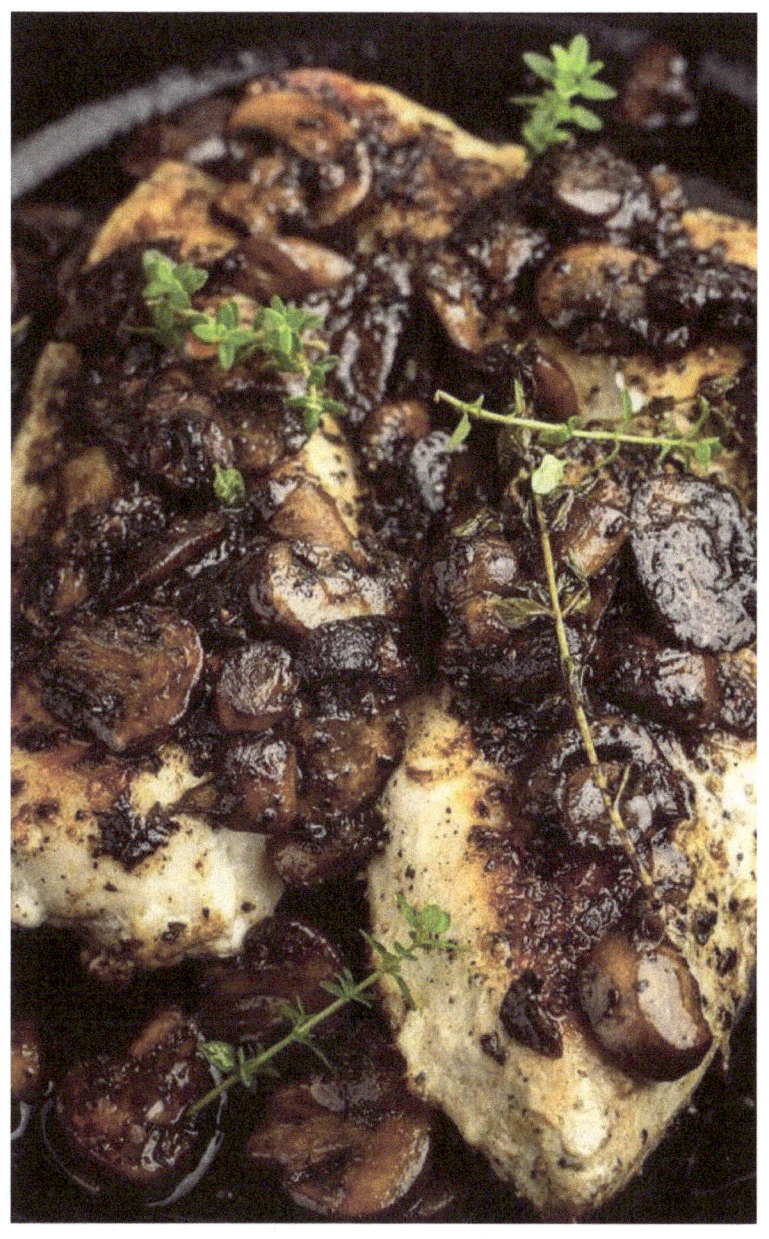

Preparation Time: 10 minutes

Cooking Time: 15 minutes

Servings: 6

Ingredients:

- 2 chicken breasts
- 1 cup of sliced white champignons
- 1 cup of sliced green chilies
- 1/2 cup of scallions; hacked
- 1 teaspoon of chopped garlic
- 1 cup of low-fat cheddar shredded cheese (1-1.5 lb. grams fat / ounce)
- 1 tablespoon of olive oil
- 1 tablespoon of butter

Directions:

1. Fry the chicken breasts with olive oil.
2. Add salt and pepper as needed.
3. Grill breasts of chicken in a plate with grill.
4. For every serving, weigh 4 ounces of chicken. (Make two servings, save leftovers for an additional meal).

5. In a butter pan, stir in mushrooms, green peppers, scallions, and garlic until smooth, and a bit dark.
6. Place the chicken in a baking platter.
7. Cover with mushroom combination.
8. Top with ham.
9. Place the cheese in a 350° F oven until it melts.

Nutrition:

- Carbohydrates: 2 g
- Protein: 23 g
- Fat: 11 g
- Cholesterol: 112 mg
- Sodium: 198 mg
- Potassium: 261 mg

Marinated Eggs

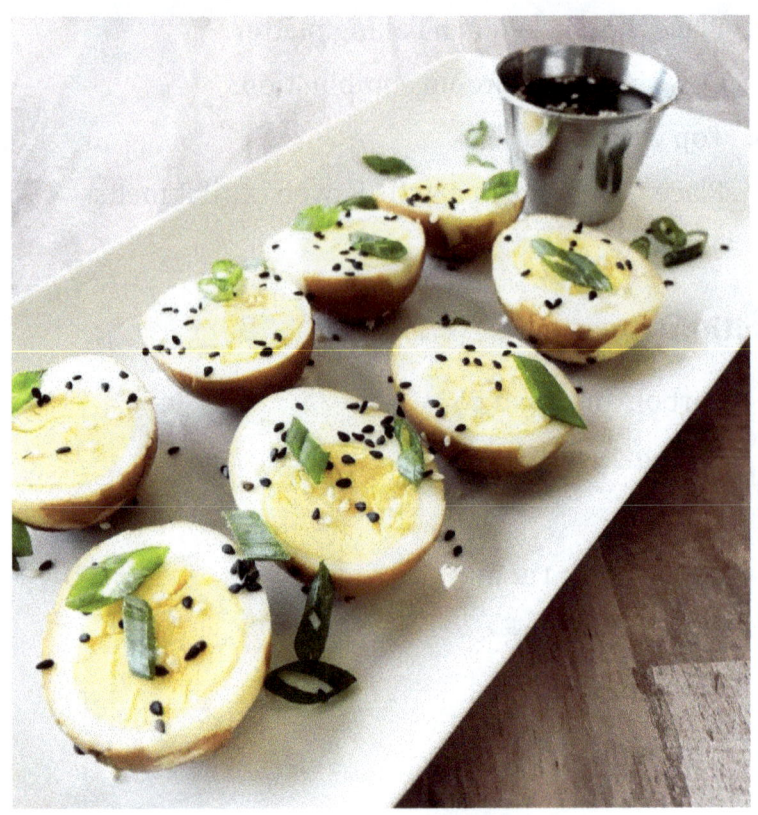

Preparation Time: 2 hours and 10 minutes

Cooking Time: 7 minutes

Servings: 4

Ingredients:

- 6 eggs

- 1 and ¼ cups of water
- ¼ cup of unsweetened rice vinegar
- 2 tablespoons of coconut aminos
- Salt and black pepper to the taste
- 2 garlic cloves; minced
- 1 teaspoon of stevia
- 4 ounces of cream cheese
- 1 tablespoon of chives; chopped

Directions:

1. Put the eggs in a pot, add water to cover, bring to a boil over medium heat, cover and cook for 7 minutes.
2. Rinse eggs with cold water and set them aside to chill down.
3. In a bowl, mix one cup of water with coconut aminos, vinegar, stevia, garlic, and whisk well.
4. Put the eggs in this mix, cover with a kitchen towel, and put them aside for 2 hours, turning from time to time.
5. Peel eggs, cut in halves, and put egg yolks in a bowl.
6. Add ¼ cup water, cream cheese, salt, pepper, chives, and stir well.

7. Stuff egg whites with this mix and serve them.
8. Enjoy!

Nutrition:

- Calories: 289
- Protein: 15.86 g
- Fat: 22.62 g
- Carbohydrates: 4.52 g
- Sodium: 288 mg

Lamb Stuffed Avocado

Preparation Time: 10 minutes

Cooking Time: 40 minutes

Servings: 4

Ingredients:

- 2 avocados
- 1 1/2 cup of minced lamb
- 1/2 cup of cheddar cheese; grated
- 1/2 cup of parmesan cheese; grated
- 2 tbsps. of almond; chopped
- 1 tbsp. of coriander; chopped
- 2 tbsps. of olive oil
- 1 tomato; chopped
- 1 jalapeno; chopped
- Salt and pepper to taste
- 1 tsp. of garlic, chopped
- 1-inch ginger; chopped

Directions:

1. Cut the avocados in half. Remove the pit and scoop out some flesh so as to be able to stuff it later.
2. In a skillet, add half the oil.
3. Toss the ginger, garlic for 1 minute.
4. Add the lamb and toss for 3 minutes.
5. Add the tomato, coriander, parmesan, jalapeno, salt, pepper, and cook for 2 minutes.
6. Take off the heat. Stuff the avocados.
7. Sprinkle the almonds, cheddar cheese, and add olive oil on top.
8. Add to a baking sheet and bake for 30 minutes. Serve.

Nutrition:

- Fat: 19.5 g
- Cholesterol: 167.5 mg
- Sodium: 410.7 mg
- Potassium: 617.1 mg
- Carbohydrate: 13.1 g

Chili Mango and Watermelon Salsa

Preparation Time: 5 minutes

Cooking Time: 0 minutes

Servings: 12

Ingredients:

- 1 red tomato; chopped
- Salt and black pepper to the taste
- 1 cup of watermelon; seedless, peeled and cubed
- 1 red onion; chopped
- 2 mangos; peeled and chopped
- 2 chili peppers; chopped
- ¼ cup of cilantro; chopped
- 3 tablespoons of lime juice
- Pita chips for serving

Directions:

1. In a bowl, mix the tomato with the watermelon, the onion, and the rest of the ingredients except the pita chips, and toss well.

2. Divide the mix into small cups and serve with pita chips on the side.

Nutrition:

- Calories: 62
- Fat: 4 g
- Fiber: 1.3 g
- Carbs: 3.9 g
- Protein: 2.3 g

Pumpkin Muffins

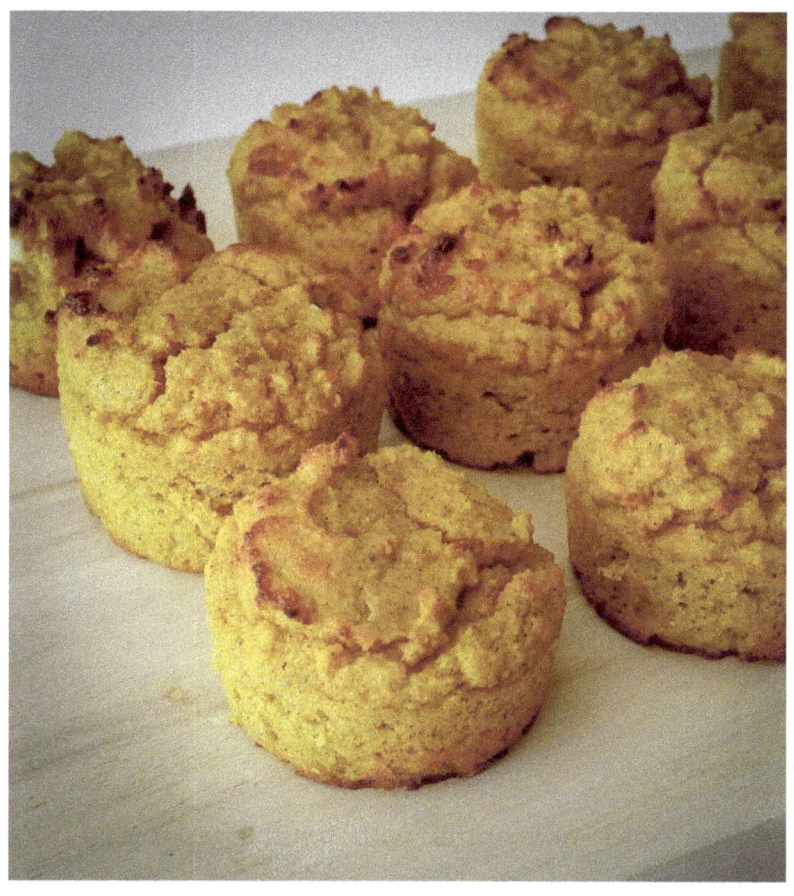

Preparation Time: 10 minutes

Cooking Time: 15 minutes

Servings: 18

Ingredients:

- ¼ cup of sunflower seed butter
- ¾ cup of pumpkin puree
- 2 tablespoons of flaxseed meal
- ¼ cup of coconut flour
- ½ cup of erythritol
- ½ teaspoon of nutmeg; ground
- 1 teaspoon of cinnamon; ground
- ½ teaspoon of baking soda
- 1 egg ½ teaspoon of baking powder
- A pinch of salt

Directions:

1. In a bowl, mix butter with pumpkin puree and egg and blend well.
2. Add flaxseed meal, coconut flour, erythritol, baking soda, baking powder, nutmeg, cinnamon, a pinch of salt, and stir well.
3. Spoon this into a greased muffin pan, put in the oven at 350º F and bake for 15 minutes.

4. Leave muffins to chill down and serve them as a snack.
5. Enjoy!

Nutrition:

- Calories: 65
- Protein: 2.82 g
- Fat: 5.42 g
- Carbohydrates: 2.27 g
- Sodium: 57 mg

Chicken Enchilada Bake

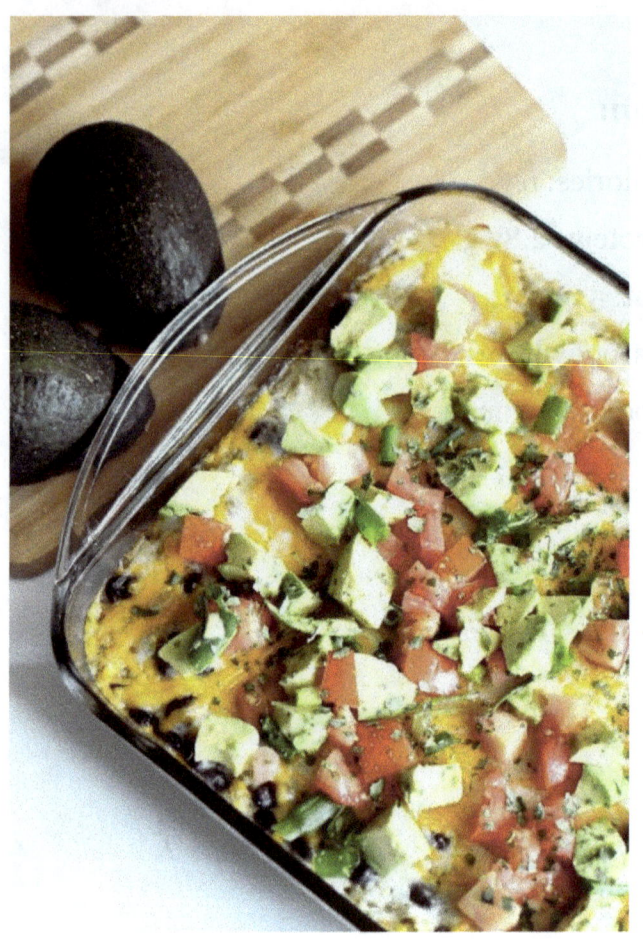

Preparation Time: 20 minutes

Cooking Time: 50 minutes

Servings: 5

Ingredients:

- 5 oz. of Shredded chicken breast (boil and shred ahead) or 99 percent fat-free white chicken can be used in a pan.
- 1 can of tomato paste
- 1 low sodium chicken broth can be fat-free
- 1/4 cup of cheese with low fat mozzarella
- 1 tablespoon of oil
- 1 tbsp. of salt
- Ground cumin, chili powder, garlic powder, oregano, and onion powder (all to taste)
- 1 to 2 zucchinis sliced vertically (similar to lasagna noodles) into thin lines
- Sliced (optional) olives

Directions:

1. Add vegetable oil in sauce pan over medium-high heat, stir in ingredients and seasonings, and heat in chicken stock for 2-3 min.
2. Turn heat to low for 15 min, stirring regularly to boil.
3. Set aside and cool to ambient temperature.
4. Pull-strip of zucchini through enchilada sauce and lay flat on the pan's bottom in a small baking pan.

5. Next, add the chicken with the 1/4 cup of enchilada sauce and blend it.
6. Place chicken to the end to end duvet of the baking tray.
7. Sprinkle some bacon over the chicken.
8. Add another layer of the pulled zucchini via enchilada sauce (similar to lasagna making).
9. When needed, cover with the remaining cheese and olives on top. Bake for 35 to 40 minutes.
10. Keep an eye on them.
11. When the cheese starts getting golden, cover with foil.
12. Serve and enjoy!

Nutrition:

- Calories: 312
- Carbohydrates: 21.3 g
- Protein: 27 g
- Fat: 10.2 g

Greek Tuna Salad Bites

Preparation Time: 5 Minutes

Cooking Time: 10 Minutes

Servings: 6

Ingredients:

- Cucumbers (2 medium)
- White tuna (2 - 6 oz. cans)
- Lemon juice (half of 1 lemon)
- Red bell pepper (.5 cup)
- Sweet/red onion (.25 cup)
- Black olives (.25 cup)
- Garlic (2 tablespoons)
- Olive oil (2 tablespoons)
- Fresh parsley (2 tablespoons)
- Dried oregano
- salt & pepper (as desired)

Directions:

1. Drain and flake the tuna. Juice the lemon. Dice/chop the onions, olives, pepper, parsley, and garlic. Slice each of the cucumbers into thick rounds (skin off or on).
2. In a mixing container, mix the rest of the ingredients.
3. Place a heaping spoonful of salad onto the rounds and enjoy.

Nutrition:

- Calories: 400
- Fats: 22 g
- Carbs: 26 g
- Fiber Content: 8 g
- Protein: 30 g

Veggie Fritters

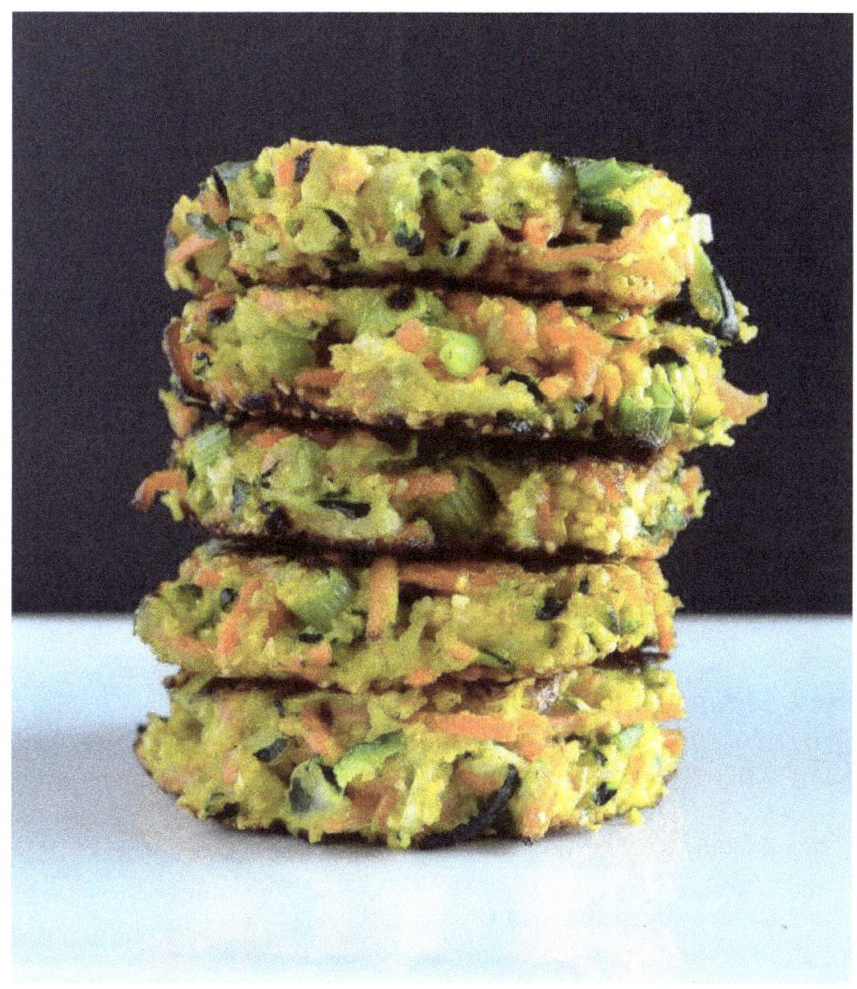

Cooking Time: 10 minutes

Servings: 4

Ingredients:

- 2 garlic cloves; minced
- 2 yellow onions; chopped
- 4 scallions; chopped
- 2 carrots; grated
- 2 teaspoons of cumin; ground
- ½ teaspoon of turmeric powder
- Salt and black pepper to the taste
- ¼ teaspoon of coriander; ground
- 2 tablespoons of parsley; chopped
- ¼ teaspoon of lemon juice
- ½ cup of almond flour
- 2 beets; peeled and grated
- 2 eggs; whisked
- ¼ cup of tapioca flour
- 3 tablespoons of olive oil

Directions:

1. In a bowl, combine the garlic with the onions, scallions, and the rest of the ingredients except the oil. Stir well and shape medium fritters out of this mix.
2. Heat up a pan with the oil over medium-high heat, add the fritters, cook for 5 minutes on all sides, arrange on a platter and serve.

Nutrition:

- Calories: 209
- Fat: 11.2 g
- Fiber: 3 g
- Carbs: 4.4 g
- Protein: 4.8 g

Olives and Cheese Stuffed Tomatoes

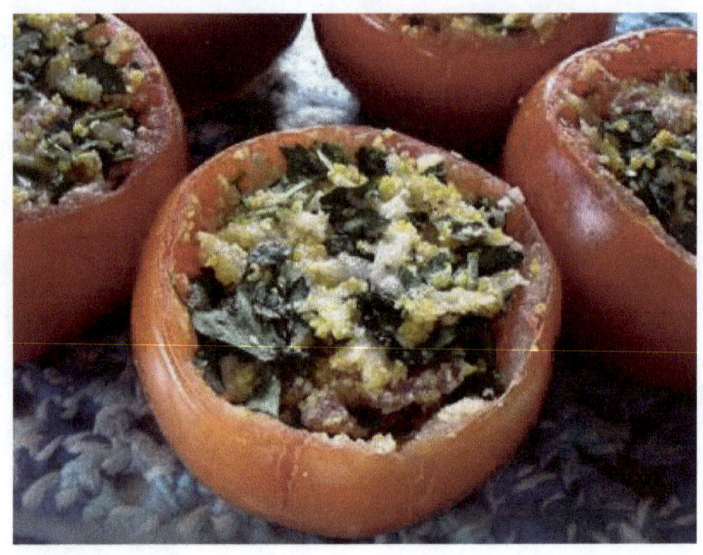

Preparation Time: 10 minutes

Cooking Time: 0 minutes

Servings: 24

Ingredients:

- 24 cherry tomatoes; top cut off and insides scooped out
- 2 tablespoons of olive oil
- ¼ teaspoon of red pepper flakes
- ½ cup of feta cheese; crumbled

- 2 tablespoons of black olive paste
- ¼ cup of mint; torn

Directions:

1. In a bowl, mix the olives paste with the rest of the ingredients except the cherry tomatoes, and whisk well.
2. Stuff the cherry tomatoes with this mix, arrange them all on a platter and serve as an appetizer.

Nutrition:

- Calories: 136
- Fat: 8.6 g
- Fiber: 4.8 g
- Carbs: 5.6 g
- Protein: 5.1 g

Cucumber Sandwich Bites

Preparation Time: 5 minutes

Cooking Time: 0 minutes

Servings: 12

Ingredients:

- 1 cucumber; sliced
- 8 slices of whole wheat bread
- 2 tablespoons of cream cheese; soft
- 1 tablespoon of chives; chopped
- ¼ cup of avocado; peeled, pitted and mashed
- 1 teaspoon of mustard
- Salt and black pepper to the taste

Directions:

1. Spread the mashed avocado on each bread slice, also spread the rest of the ingredients except the cucumber slices.

2. Divide the cucumber slices on the bread slices, cut each slice in thirds, arrange on a platter and serve as an appetizer.

Nutrition:

- Calories: 187
- Fat: 12.4 g
- Fiber: 2.1 g
- Carbs: 4.5 g
- Protein 8.2 g

White Bean Dip

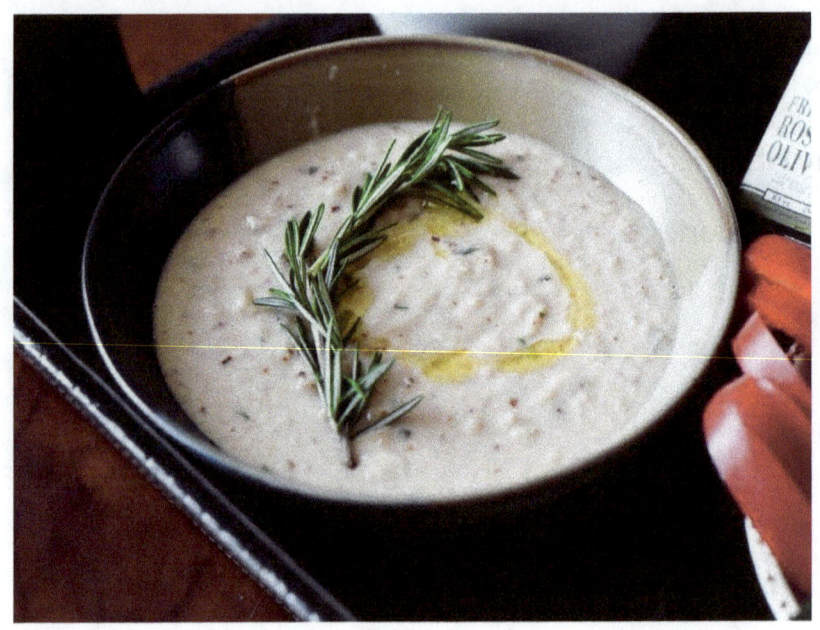

Cooking Time: 0 minute

Servings: 4

Ingredients:

- 15 ounces of canned white beans; drained and rinsed
- 6 ounces of canned artichoke hearts; drained and quartered
- 4 garlic cloves; minced

- 1 tablespoon of basil; chopped
- 2 tablespoons of olive oil
- Juice of ½ lemon
- Zest of ½ lemon; grated
- Salt and black pepper to the taste

Directions:

1. In your food processor, mix the beans with the artichokes and the rest of the ingredients except the oil and pulse well.
2. Add the oil gradually, pulse the combination again, divide into cups and serve with a celebration dip.

Nutrition:

- Calories: 274
- Fat: 11.7 g
- Fiber: 6.5 g
- Carbs: 18.5 g
- Protein: 16.5 g

Eggplant Dip

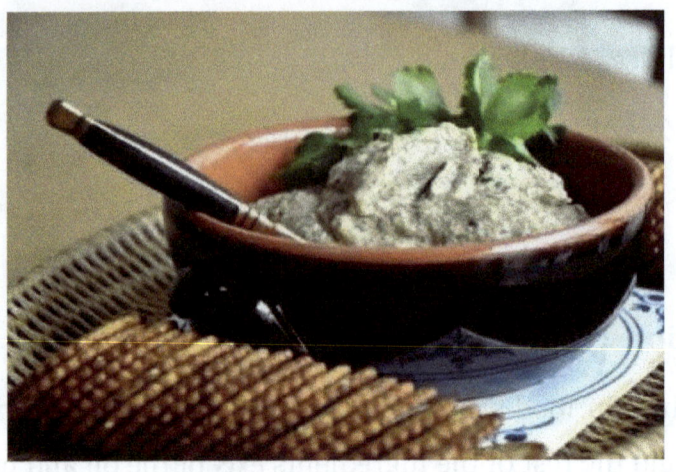

Cooking Time: 40 minutes

Servings: 4

Ingredients:

- 1 eggplant; poked with a fork
- 2 tablespoons of tahini paste
- 2 tablespoons of lemon juice
- 2 garlic cloves; minced
- 1 tablespoon of olive oil
- Salt and black pepper to the taste

- 1 tablespoon of parsley; chopped

Directions:

1. Put the eggplant in a roasting pan, bake at 400°F for 40 minutes, allow to cool down, then peel and transfer to your food processor.
2. Add the rest of the ingredients except the parsley, pulse well, divide into small bowls and serve an appetizer with the parsley sprinkled on top.

Nutrition:

- Calories: 121
- Fat: 4.3 g
- Fiber: 1 g
- Carbs: 1.4 g
- Protein: 4.3 g

Tomato Salsa

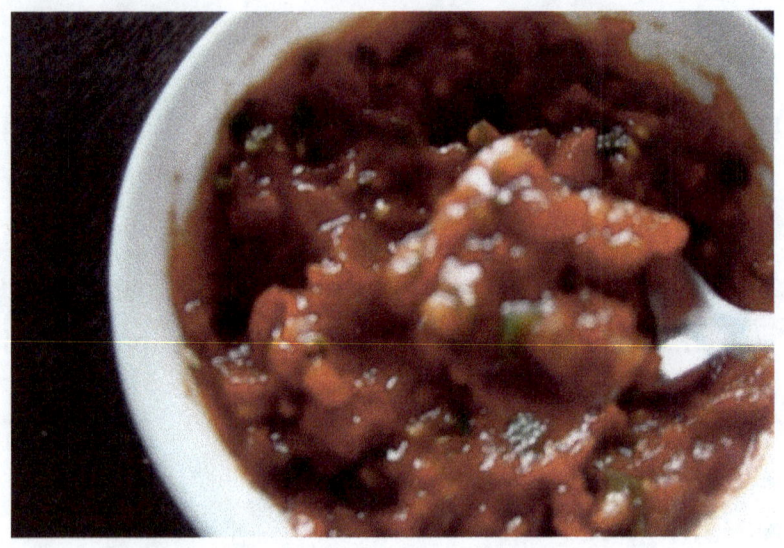

Preparation Time: 5 minutes

Cooking Time: 0 minutes

Servings: 6

Ingredients:

- 1 garlic clove; minced
- 4 tablespoons of olive oil
- 5 tomatoes; cubed
- 1 tablespoon of balsamic vinegar

- ¼ cup of basil; chopped
- 1 tablespoon of parsley; chopped
- 1 tablespoon of chives; chopped
- Salt and black pepper to the taste
- Pita chips for serving

Directions:

In a bowl, mix the tomatoes with the garlic and the rest of the ingredients except the pita chips, stir, divide into small cups and serve with the pita chips on the side.

Nutrition:

- Calories: 160
- Fat: 13.7 g
- Fiber: 5.5 g
- Carbs: 10.1 g
- Protein: 2.2 g

Feta Artichoke Dip

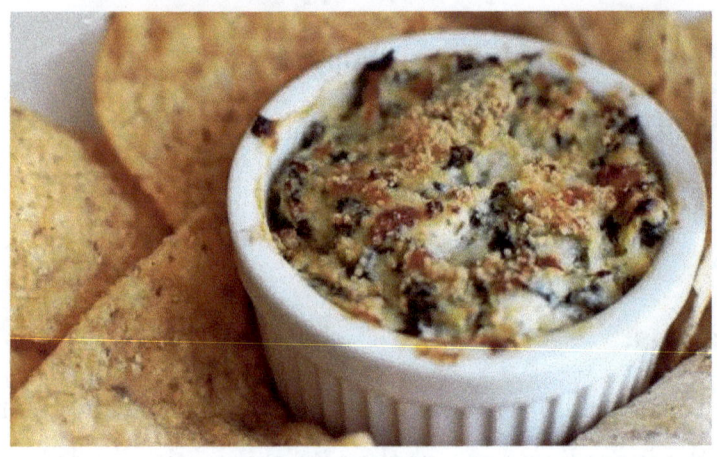

Preparation Time: 10 minutes

Cooking Time: 30 minutes

Servings: 8

Ingredients:

- 8 ounces of artichoke hearts; drained and quartered
- ¾ cup of basil; chopped
- ¾ cup of green olives; pitted and chopped
- 1 cup of parmesan cheese; grated
- 5 ounces of feta cheese; crumbled

Directions:

1. In your food processor, mix the artichokes with the basil and the rest of the ingredients, pulse well, and transfer to a baking dish.
2. Put in the oven, bake at 375°F for 30 minutes and serve as a party dip.

Nutrition:

- Calories: 186
- Fat: 12.4 g
- Fiber: 0.9 g
- Carbs: 2.6 g
- Protein: 1.5 g

Bulgur Lamb Meatballs

Preparation Time: 10 minutes

Cooking Time: 15 minute

Servings: 6

Ingredients:

- 1 ½ cups of Greek yogurt
- ½ teaspoon of cumin; ground
- 1 cup of cucumber; shredded
- ½ teaspoon of garlic; minced
- A pinch of salt and black pepper
- 1 cup of bulgur
- 2 cups of water
- 1 pound of lamb; ground
- ¼ cup of parsley; chopped
- ¼ cup of shallots; chopped
- ½ teaspoon of allspice; ground
- ½ teaspoon of cinnamon powder
- 1 tablespoon of olive oil

Directions:

1. In a bowl, mix the bulgur with the water, cover the bowl, put aside for 10 minutes, drain and transfer to a bowl.
2. Add the meat, the yogurt and the rest of the ingredients except the oil, stir well and shape medium meatballs out of the mix.
3. Heat up a pan with the oil over medium-high heat, add the meatballs, cook them for 7 minutes on all sides, arrange all of them on a platter and serve as an appetizer.

Nutrition:

- Calories: 300
- Fat: 9.6 g
- Fiber: 4.6 g
- Carbs: 22.6 g
- Protein: 6.6 g

Cucumber Bites

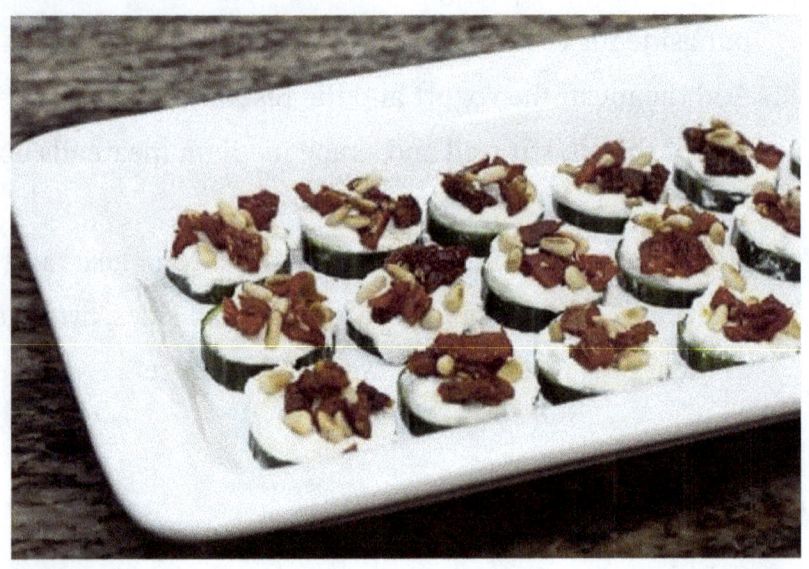

Preparation Time: 10 minutes

Cooking Time: 0 minutes

Servings: 12

Ingredients:

- 1 English cucumber; sliced into 32 rounds
- 10 ounces of hummus
- 16 cherry tomatoes; halved
- 1 tablespoon of parsley; chopped

- 1 ounce of feta cheese; crumbled

Directions:

Spread the hummus on each cucumber round, divide the tomato halves on each, sprinkle the cheese and parsley on top and serve as an appetizer.

Nutrition:

- Calories: 162
- Fat: 3.4 g
- Fiber: 2 g
- Carbs: 6.4 g
- Protein: 2.4 g

Hummus with Ground Lamb

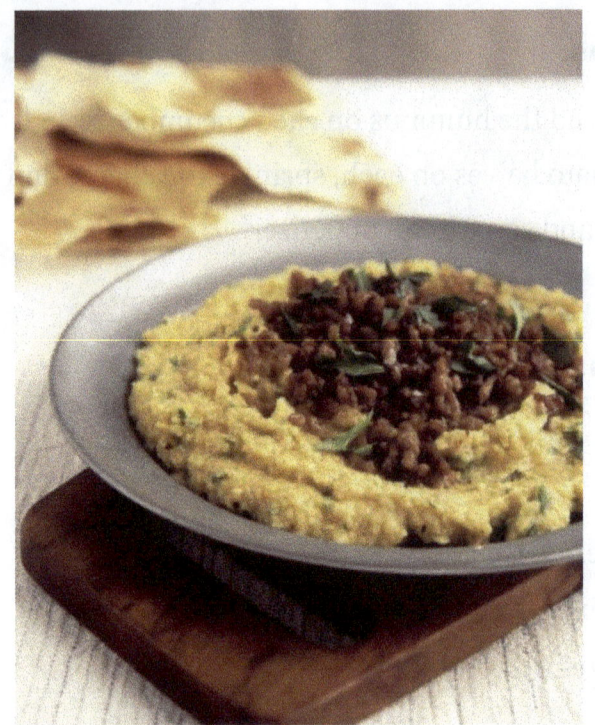

Preparation Time: 10 minutes

Cooking Time: 15 minutes

Servings: 8

Ingredients:

- 10 ounces of hummus
- 12 ounces of lamb meat; ground

- ½ cup of pomegranate seeds
- ¼ cup of parsley; chopped
- 1 tablespoon of olive oil
- Pita chips for serving

Directions:
1. Heat up a pan with the oil over medium-high heat, add the meat, and brown for 15 minutes stirring often.
2. Spread the hummus on a platter, spread the ground lamb all over, also spread the pomegranate seeds and the parsley and serve with pita chips as a snack.

Nutrition:
- Calories: 133
- Fat: 9.7 g
- Fiber: 1.7 g
- Carbs: 6.4 g
- Protein: 5 g

Wrapped Plums

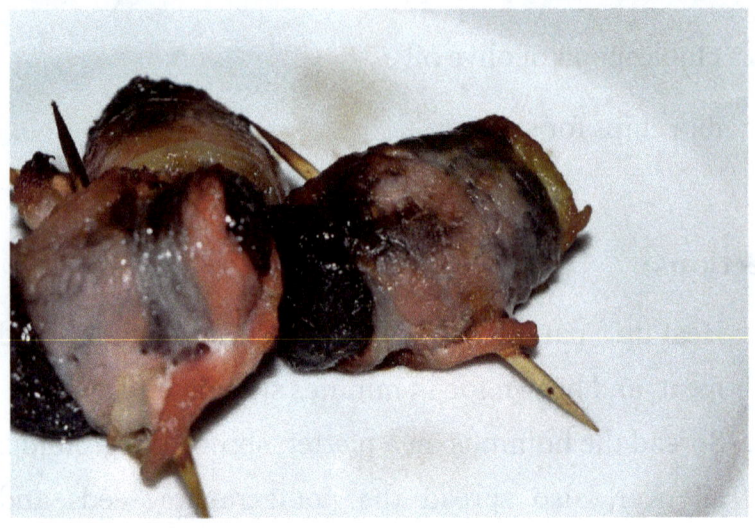

Preparation Time: 5 minutes

Cooking Time: 0 minutes

Servings: 8

Ingredients:

- 2 ounces of prosciutto; cut into 16 pieces
- 4 plums; quartered
- 1 tablespoon of chives; chopped
- A pinch of red pepper flakes; crushed

Directions:

Wrap each plum quarter in a prosciutto slice, arrange them all on a platter, sprinkle the chives and pepper flakes all over and serve.

Nutrition:

- Calories: 30
- Fat: 1 g
- Fiber: 0 g
- Carbs: 4 g
- Protein: 2 g

Cucumber Rolls

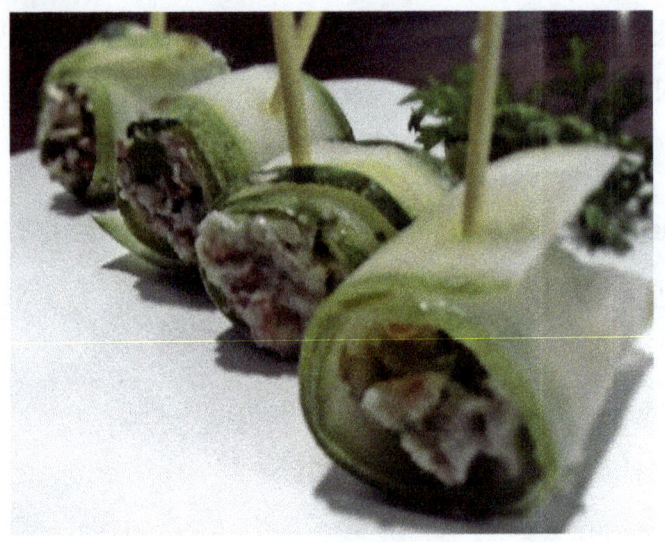

Preparation Time: 5 minutes

Cooking Time: 0 minutes

Servings: 6

Ingredients:

- 1 big cucumber; sliced lengthwise
- 1 tablespoon of parsley; chopped
- 8 ounces of canned tuna; drained and mashed
- Salt and black pepper to the taste

- 1 teaspoon of lime juice

Directions:

1. Arrange cucumber slices on a working surface, divide the rest of the ingredients among the slices, and roll.
2. Arrange all the rolls on a platter and serve as an appetizer.

Nutrition:

- Calories: 200
- Fat: 6 g
- Fiber: 3.4 g
- Carbs: 7.6 g
- Protein: 3.5 g

Creamy Spinach and Shallots Dip

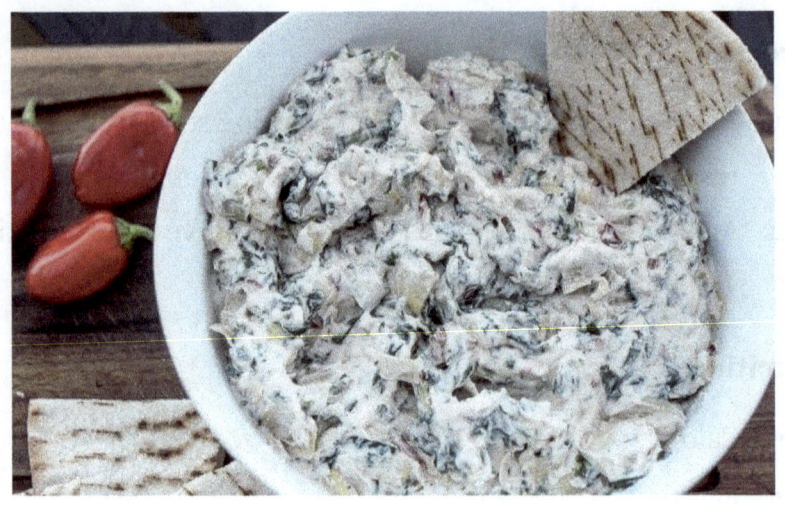

Preparation Time: 10 minutes

Cooking Time: 0 minutes

Servings: 4

Ingredients:

- 1 pound of spinach; roughly chopped
- 2 shallots; chopped
- 2 tablespoons of mint; chopped
- ¾ cup of cream cheese; soft
- Salt and black pepper to your taste

Directions:

1. In a blender, mix the spinach with the shallots and the rest of the ingredients, and pulse well.
2. Divide into small bowls and serve as a party dip.

Nutrition:

1. Calories: 204
2. Fat: 11.5 g
3. Fiber: 3.1 g
4. Carbs: 4.2 g
5. Protein: 5.9 g

Avocado Dip

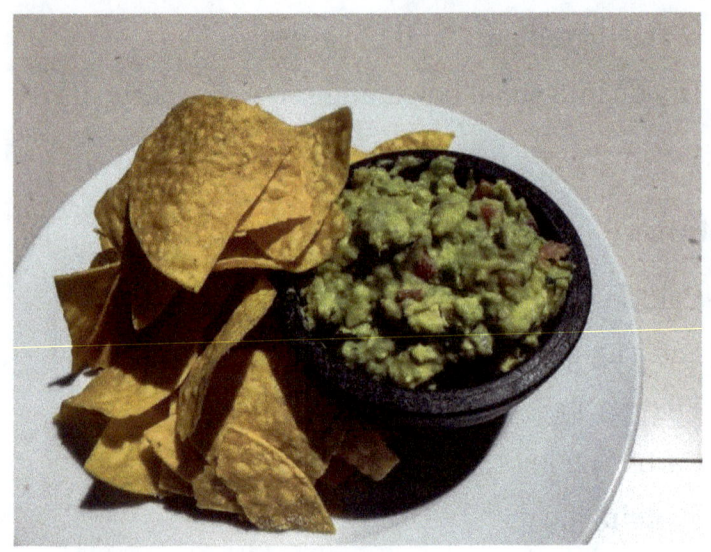

Preparation Time: 5 minutes

Cooking Time: 0 minutes

Servings: 8

Ingredients:

- ½ cup of heavy cream
- 1 green chili pepper; chopped
- Salt and pepper to the taste
- 4 avocados; pitted, peeled and chopped

- 1 cup of cilantro; chopped
- ¼ cup of lime juice

Directions:

1. In a blender, mix the cream with the avocados and the rest of the ingredients, and pulse well.
2. Divide the mix into bowls and serve cold as a party dip.

Nutrition:

- Calories: 200
- Fat: 14.5 g
- Fiber: 3.8 g
- Carbs: 8.1 g
- Protein: 7.6 g

Goat Cheese and Chives Spread

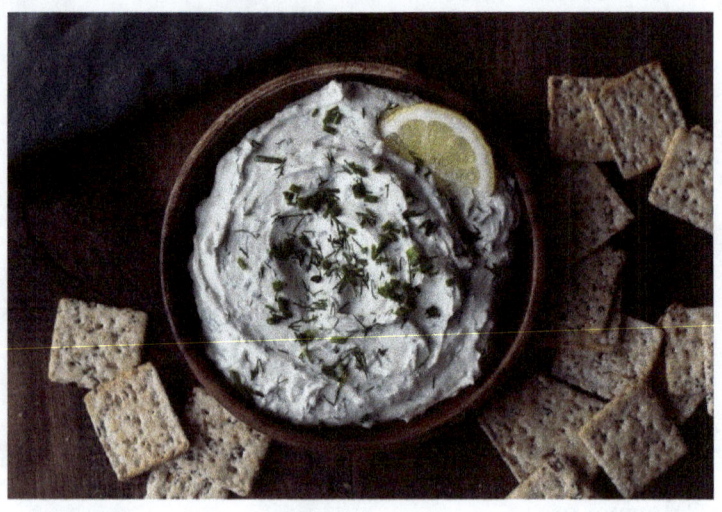

Preparation Time: 10 minutes

Cooking Time: 0 minutes

Servings: 4

Ingredients:

- 2 ounces of goat cheese; crumbled
- ¾ cup of sour cream
- 2 tablespoons of chives; chopped
- 1 tablespoon of lemon juice
- Salt and black pepper to your taste

- 2 tablespoons of extra virgin olive oil

Directions:

1. In a bowl, mix the goat cheese with the cream and the rest of the ingredients, and whisk really well.
2. Keep in the fridge for 10 minutes and serve as a party spread.

Nutrition:

- Calories: 220
- Fat: 11.5 g
- Fiber: 4.8 g
- Carbs: 8.9 g
- Protein: 5.6 g

Chia Pudding

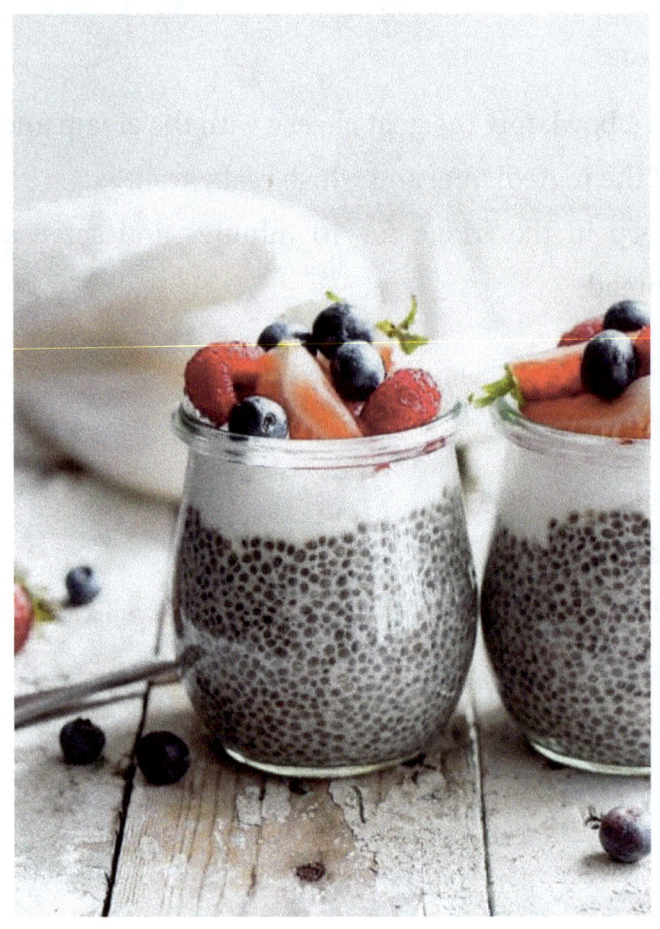

Preparation Time: 20 minutes

Cooking Time: 0 minutes

Servings: 2

Ingredients:

- 4 tbsps. of chia seeds
- 1 cup of unsweetened coconut milk
- 1/2 cup of raspberries

Directions:

1. Add raspberry and coconut milk into a blender and blend until smooth.
2. Pour mixture into the glass jar.
3. Add chia seeds in a jar and stir well.
4. Seal the jar with a lid, shake well and place in the refrigerator for 3 hours.
5. Serve chilled and enjoy.

Nutrition:

- Calories: 360
- Fat: 33 g
- Carbs: 13 g
- Sugar: 5 g
- Protein: 6 g
- Cholesterol: 0 mg

Avocado Pudding

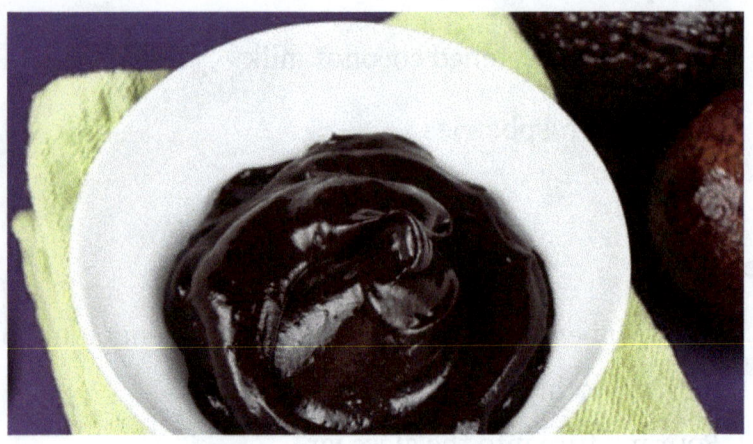

Preparation Time: 20 minutes

Cooking Time: 0 minutes

Servings: 8

Ingredients:

- 2 ripe avocados, pitted and cut into pieces
- 1 tbsps. of fresh lime juice
- 14 oz. can of coconut milk
- 2 tsps. of liquid stevia
- 2 tsps. of vanilla

Directions:

1. Inside the blender, add all ingredients and blend until smooth.
2. Serve immediately and enjoy.

Nutrition:

- Calories: 317
- Fat: 30 g
- Carbs: 9 g
- Sugar: 0.5 g
- Protein: 3 g
- Cholesterol: 0 mg

Smooth Peanut Butter Cream

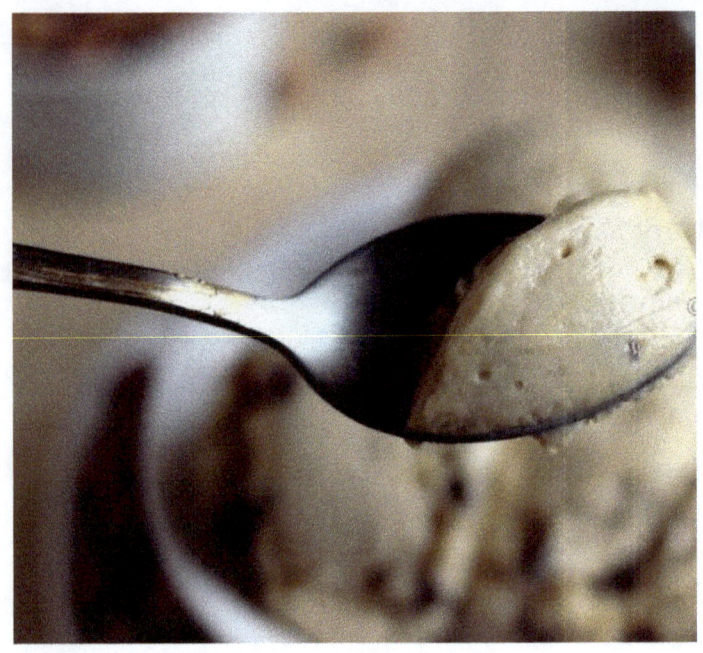

Preparation Time: 10 minutes

Cooking Time: 0 minutes

Servings: 8

Ingredients:

- 1/4 cup of peanut butter
- 4 overripe bananas; chopped
- 1/3 cup of cocoa powder

- 1/4 tsp. of vanilla extract
- 1/8 tsp. of salt

Directions:

1. Add all the listed ingredients in a blender and blend until smooth.
2. Serve immediately and enjoy.

Nutrition:

- Calories: 101
- Fat: 5 g
- Carbs: 14 g
- Sugar: 7 g
- Protein: 3 g
- Cholesterol: 0 mg

Raspberry Ice Cream

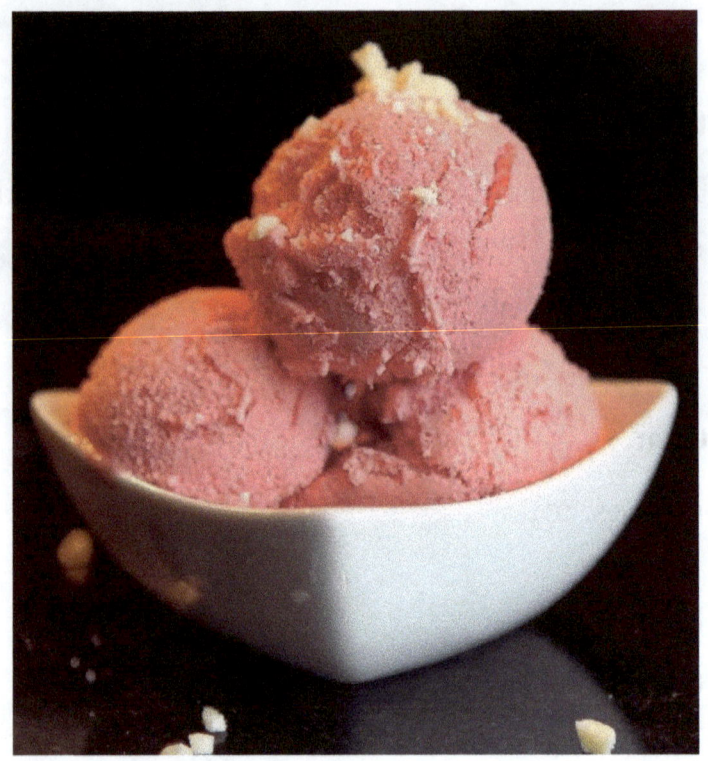

Preparation Time: 10 minutes

Servings: 2

Ingredients:

- 1 cup of frozen raspberries
- 1/2 cup of heavy cream

- 1/8 tsp. of stevia powder

Directions:

1. Blend all the listed ingredients in a blender until smooth.
2. Serve immediately and enjoy.

Nutrition:

- Calories: 144
- Fat: 11 g
- Carbs: 10 g
- Sugar: 4 g
- Protein: 2 g
- Cholesterol: 41 mg

Chocolate Frosty

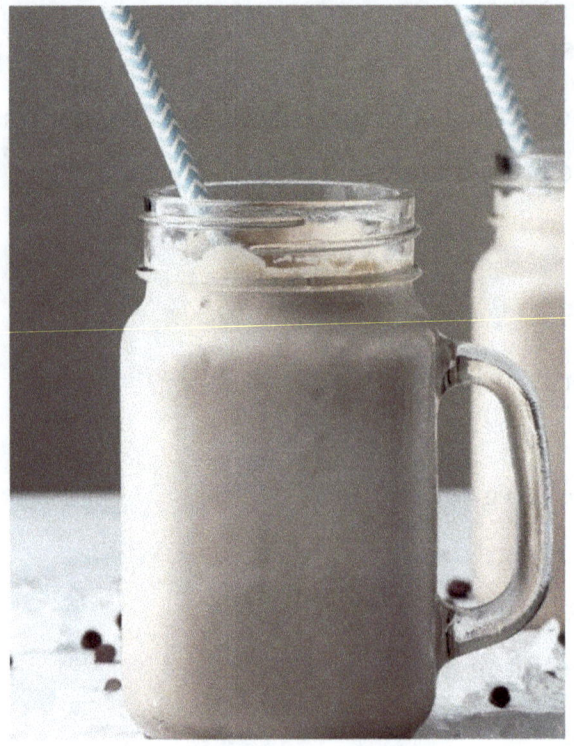

Preparation Time: 20 minutes

Cooking Time: 0 minutes

Servings: 4

Ingredients:

- 2 tbsps. of unsweetened cocoa powder
- 1 cup of heavy whipping cream

- 1 tbsp. of almond butter
- 5 drops of liquid stevia
- 1 tsp. of vanilla

Directions:

1. Add cream into a medium bowl and beat using the hand mixer for 5 minutes.
2. Add the remaining ingredients and blend until a thick cream forms.
3. Pour in serving bowls and place them in the freezer for 30 minutes.
4. Serve and enjoy.

Nutrition:

- Calories: 137
- Fat: 13 g
- Carbs: 3 g
- Sugar: 0.5 g
- Protein: 2 g
- Cholesterol: 41 mg

Cranberry Muffins

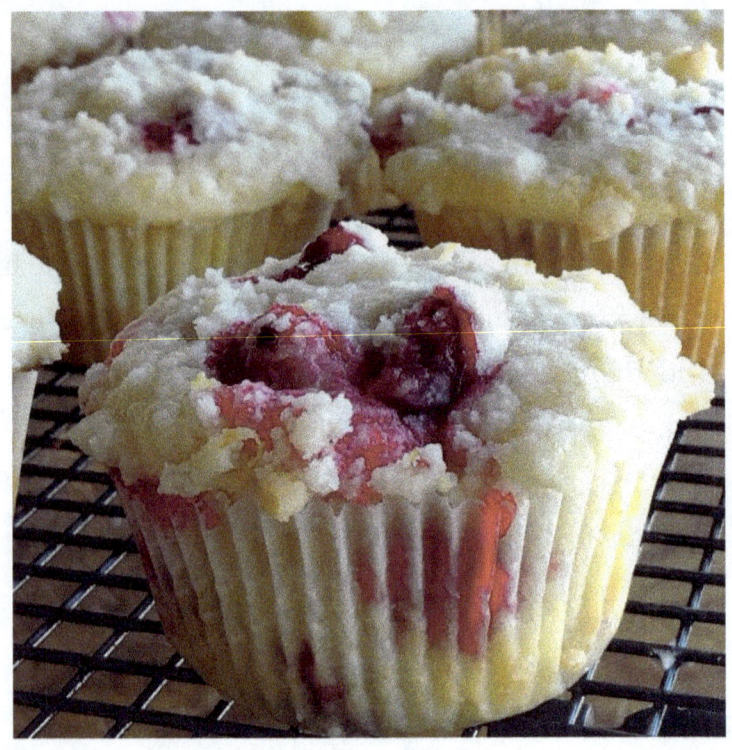

Servings: 8

Preparation Time: 25 minutes

Cooking Time: 15 minutes

Ingredients:

- ¼ cup of unsweetened almond milk
- 2 large eggs

- ½ teaspoon of vanilla extract
- 1½ cups of almond flour
- ¼ cup of Erythritol
- 1 teaspoon of baking powder
- ¼ teaspoon of ground cinnamon
- 1/8 teaspoon of salt
- ½ cup of fresh cranberries
- ¼ cup of walnuts, chopped

Instructions:

1. In a blender, add the almond milk, eggs, vanilla, and pulse for about 20-30 seconds.
2. Add the almond flour, Erythritol, baking powder, cinnamon, salt, and pulse for about 30-45 seconds until well blended.
3. Transfer the mixture into a bowl.
4. Gently fold in half the cranberries and walnuts.
5. Place the mixture into 8 silicone muffin cups of and top each with remaining cranberries.
6. Select "Air Fry" of Breville Smart Air Fryer Oven and adjust the temperature to 325 degrees F.
7. Set the timer for 15 minutes and press "Start/Stop" to start preheating.

8. When the unit beeps to point out that it's preheated, arrange the muffin cups of over the wire rack.
9. When the cooking time is completed, remove the muffin cups of from oven and place onto a wire rack to chill for about 10 minutes.
10. Carefully invert the muffins onto the wire rack to completely cool before serving.

Bounty Bars

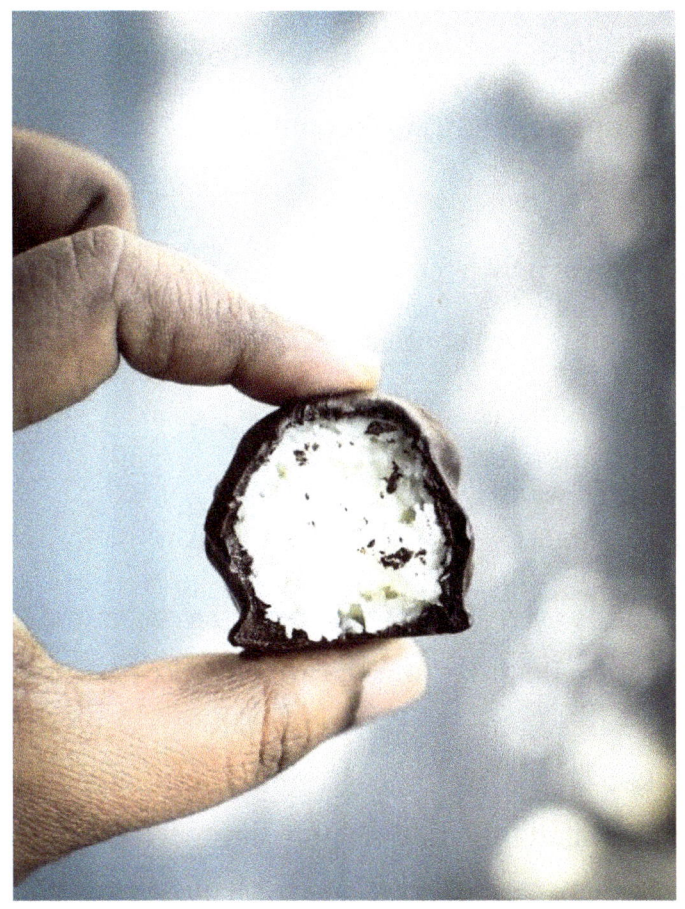

Preparation Time: 20 minutes

Cooking Time: 0 minutes

Servings: 12

Ingredients:

- 1 cup of coconut cream
- 3 cups of shredded unsweetened coconut
- 1/4 cup of extra virgin coconut oil
- 1/2 teaspoon of vanilla powder
- 1/4 cup of powdered erythritol
- 1 1/2 oz. of cocoa butter
- 5 oz. of dark chocolate

Directions:

1. Heat the oven at 350°F and toast the coconut in it for 5-6 minutes. Remove from the oven once toasted and put aside to cool.
2. Take a bowl of medium size and add coconut oil, coconut milk, vanilla, erythritol, and toasted coconut. Mix the ingredients well to form a smooth mixture.
3. With your hands, make 12 bars of equal size from the prepared mixture and adjust in the tray lined with parchment paper.
4. Place the tray in the fridge for about 1 hour and, in the meantime, put the cocoa butter and dark chocolate in a glass bowl.

5. Heat a cup of water in a saucepan over medium heat and place the bowl over it to melt the cocoa butter and the dark chocolate.
6. Remove from the heat once melted properly, mix well until blended and put aside to cool.
7. Take the coconut bars and coat them with dark chocolate mixture one by one using a wooden stick. Adjust on the tray lined with parchment paper and drizzle the remaining mixture over them.
8. Refrigerate for around 1 hour before you serve the delicious bounty bars.

Nutrition:

- Calories: 230
- Fat: 25 g
- Carbohydrates: 5 g
- Protein: 32 g

Delicious Brownie Bites

Preparation Time: 20 minutes

Cooking Time: 0 minutes

Servings: 13

Ingredients:

- 1/4 cup of unsweetened chocolate chips
- 1/4 cup of unsweetened cocoa powder
- 1 cup of pecans; chopped
- 1/2 cup of almond butter
- 1/2 tsp. of vanilla
- 1/4 cup of monk fruit sweetener
- 1/8 tsp. of pink salt

Directions:

1. Add pecans, sweetener, vanilla, almond butter, cocoa powder, and salt into the food processor and process until well mixed.
2. Transfer brownie mixture into the massive bowl. Add chocolate chips and fold well.

3. Make small sized balls from the brownie mixture and place onto a baking tray.
4. Place in the freezer for 20 minutes.
5. Serve and enjoy.

Nutrition:

- Calories: 108
- Fat: 9 g
- Carbs: 4 g
- Sugar: 1 g
- Protein: 2 g
- Cholesterol: 0 mg

Chocolate Popsicle

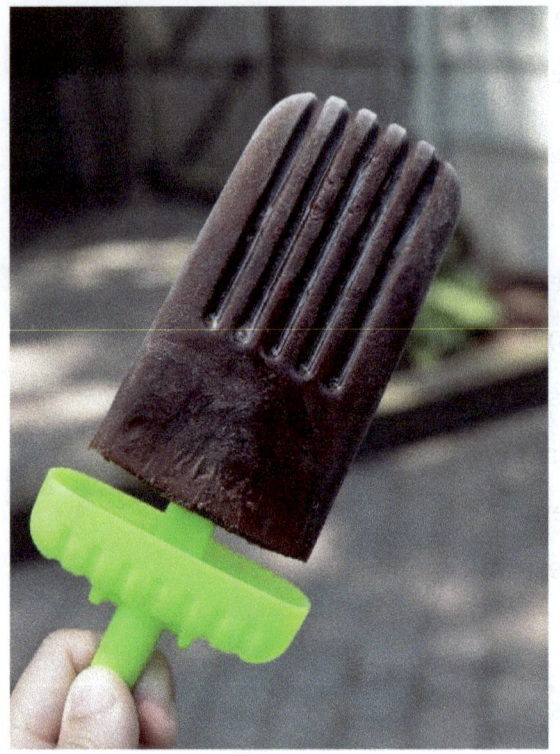

Preparation Time: 20 minutes

Cooking Time: 10 minutes

Servings: 6

Ingredients:

- 4 oz. of unsweetened chocolate; chopped

- 6 drops of liquid stevia
- 1 1/2 cups of heavy cream

Directions:

1. Add cream into the microwave-safe bowl and microwave until it just starts to boil.
2. Add chocolate into the cream and put aside for 5 minutes.
3. Add liquid stevia into the cream mixture and stir until chocolate is melted. Pour mixture into the Popsicle molds and place in freezer for 4 hours or until set.
4. Serve and enjoy.

Nutrition:

- Calories: 198
- Fat: 21 g
- Carbs: 6 g
- Sugar: 0.2 g
- Protein: 3 g
- Cholesterol: 41 mg

Pumpkin Balls

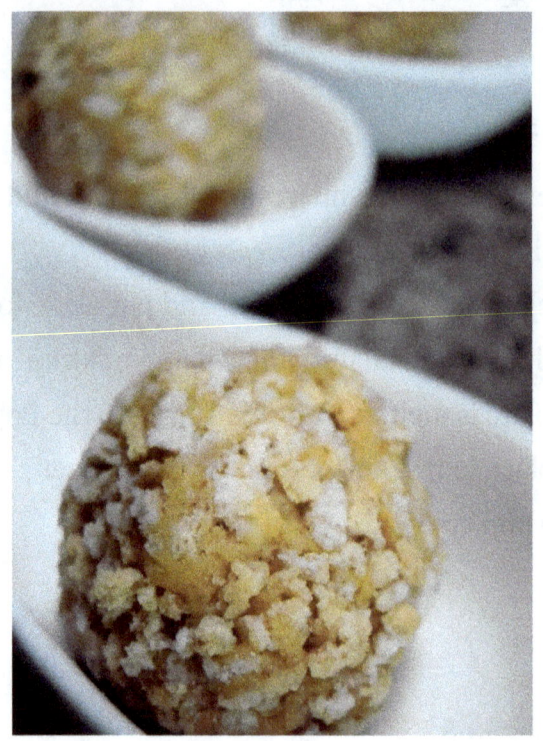

Preparation Time: 15 minutes

Cooking Time: 0 minutes

Servings: 18

Ingredients:

- 1 cup of almond butter
- 5 drops of liquid stevia

- 2 tbsps. of coconut flour
- 2 tbsps. of pumpkin puree
- 1 tsp. of pumpkin pie spice

Directions:

1. Mix together the pumpkin puree and almond butter in a large bowl, until well mixed.
2. Add liquid stevia, pie spice, coconut flour, and blend well.
3. Make small balls from the mixture and place onto a baking tray.
4. Place in the freezer for 1 hour.
5. Serve and enjoy.

Nutrition:

- Calories: 96
- Fat: 8 g
- Carbs: 4 g
- Sugar: 1 g
- Protein: 2 g
- Cholesterol: 0 mg

Blueberry Muffins

Preparation Time: 15 minutes

Cooking Time: 35 minutes

Servings: 12

Ingredients:

- 2 eggs
- 1/2 cup of fresh blueberries
- 1 cup of heavy cream
- 2 cups of almond flour
- 1/4 tsp. of lemon zest
- 1/2 tsp. of lemon extract
- 1 tsp. of baking powder
- 5 drops of stevia
- 1/4 cup of butter; melted

Directions:
1. Heat the cooker to 350 °F. Line muffin tin with cupcake liners and put aside.
2. Add eggs into the bowl and whisk until well mixed.

3. Add the remaining ingredients and blend to mix.
4. Pour mixture into the prepared muffin tin and bake for 25 minutes.
5. Serve and enjoy.

Nutrition:
- Calories: 190
- Fat: 17 g
- Carbs: 5 g
- Sugar: 1 g
- Protein: 5 g
- Cholesterol: 55 mg

Vanilla Avocado Popsicles

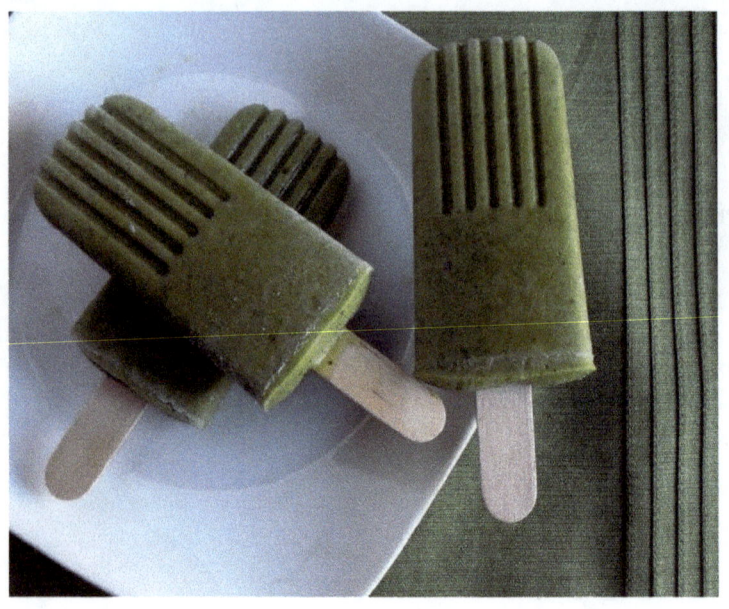

Preparation Time: 20 minutes

Cooking Time: 0 minutes

Servings: 6

Ingredients:

- 2 avocadoes
- 1 tsp. of vanilla
- 1 cup of almond milk
- 1 tsp. of liquid stevia

- 1/2 cup of unsweetened cocoa powder

Directions:

1. Add all the listed ingredients in a blender and blend until smooth.
2. Pour blended mixture into the Popsicle molds and place in the freezer until ready.
3. Serve and enjoy.

Nutrition:

- Calories: 130
- Fat: 12 g
- Carbs: 7 g
- Sugar: 1 g
- Protein: 3 g
- Cholesterol: 0 mg

Green Pea Guacamole

Preparation Time: 15 minutes

Cooking Time: 35 minutes

Servings: 4

Ingredients:

- 1 teaspoon of crushed garlic
- 1 chopped tomato
- 3 cups of frozen green peas (chopped)
- 5 green chopped onions
- 1/6 teaspoon of hot sauce
- 1/2 teaspoon of grounded cumin
- 1/2 cup of lime juice

Directions:

1. Blend the peas, garlic, lime juice, and cumin until it's smoothened.
2. Stir in the tomatoes, chopped onion, and sauce into the mixture.
3. Then add salt to taste.

4. Cover it and put it into the refrigerator for at least 30 minutes. This may allow the flavor to blend very well.

Nutrition:
- Calories: 40.7
- Fat: 0.2 g
- Cholesterol: 0.0 mg
- Sodium: 157.4 mg
- Carbohydrates: 7.6 g
- Dietary Fiber: 1.7 g
- Protein: 2.7 g

Crispy Rye Bread Snacks with Guacamole and Anchovies

Preparation time: 10 minutes

Cooking time: 10 minutes

Servings: 4

Ingredients:

- 4 slices of rye bread
- Guacamole
- Anchovies in oil

Directions:

1. Cut each slice of bread into three strips of bread.
2. Place in the basket of the air fryer without piling up and enter figures that will give it the touch you would like it to have. You can choose 180º C, 10 minutes.
3. When you have all the crusty bread strips, put a layer of guacamole on top, whether homemade or commercial.
4. In each bread, place two anchovies on the guacamole.

5. Serve and enjoy!

Nutrition:

- Calories: 180
- Carbs: 4 g
- Fat: 11 g
- Protein: 4 g
- Fiber: 9 g

Chocolate Almond Butter Brownie

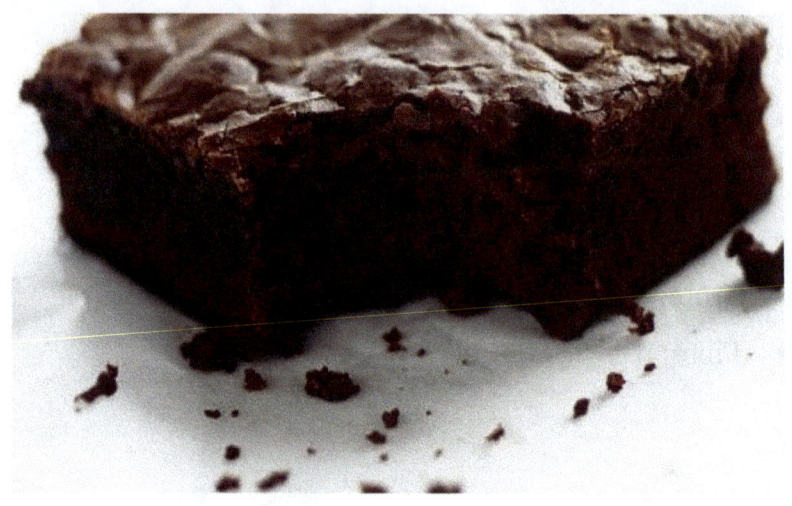

Preparation Time: 10 minutes

Cooking Time: 16 minutes

Servings: 4

Ingredients:

- 1 cup of bananas; overripe
- 1/2 cup of almond butter; melted
- 1 scoop of protein powder
- 2 tbsps. of unsweetened cocoa powder

Directions:

1. Preheat the air fryer to 325° F. Grease air fryer baking pan and set aside.
2. Blend all the ingredients in a blender until smooth.
3. Pour batter into the prepared pan and place in the air fryer basket and cook for 16 minutes.
4. Serve and enjoy.

Nutrition:

- Calories: 82
- Fat: 2 g
- Carbs: 11 g
- Sugar: 5 g
- Protein: 7 g
- Cholesterol: 16 mg

Peanut Butter Fudge

Preparation Time: 10 minutes

Cooking Time: 10 minutes

Servings: 20

Ingredients:

- 1/4 cup of almonds; toasted and chopped
- 12 oz. of smooth peanut butter
- 15 drops of liquid stevia
- 3 tbsps. of coconut oil
- 4 tbsps. of coconut cream
- Pinch of salt

Directions:

1. Line baking tray with parchment paper.
2. Melt coconut oil in a pan over low heat. Add peanut butter, coconut cream, liquid stevia, and salt in a saucepan. Stir well.
3. Pour fudge mixture into the prepared baking tray and sprinkle chopped almonds on top.

4. Place the tray in the refrigerator for 1 hour or until ready to serve.
5. Slice and serve.

Nutrition:
- Calories: 131
- Fat: 12 g
- Carbs: 4 g
- Sugar: 2 g
- Protein: 5 g
- Cholesterol: 0 mg

Almond Butter Fudge

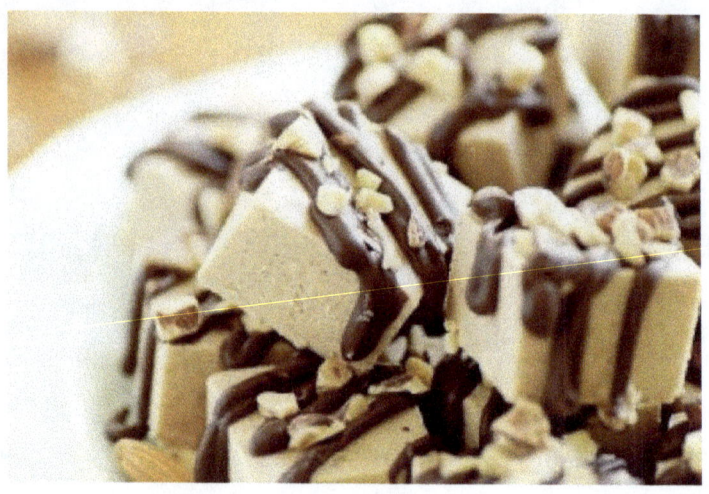

Preparation Time: 10 minutes

Cooking Time: 10 minutes

Servings: 18

Ingredients:

- 3/4 cup of creamy almond butter
- 1 1/2 cups of unsweetened chocolate chips

Directions:

1. Line 8x4-inch pan with parchment paper and put aside.

2. Add chocolate chips and almond butter into the double saucepan and cook over medium heat until the chocolate-butter mixture is melted. Stir well. Place mixture into the prepared pan and place in the freezer until ready to serve.
3. Slice and serve.

Nutrition:

- Calories: 197
- Fat: 16 g
- Carbs: 7 g
- Sugar: 1 g
- Protein: 4 g
- Cholesterol: 0 mg

Lean Granola

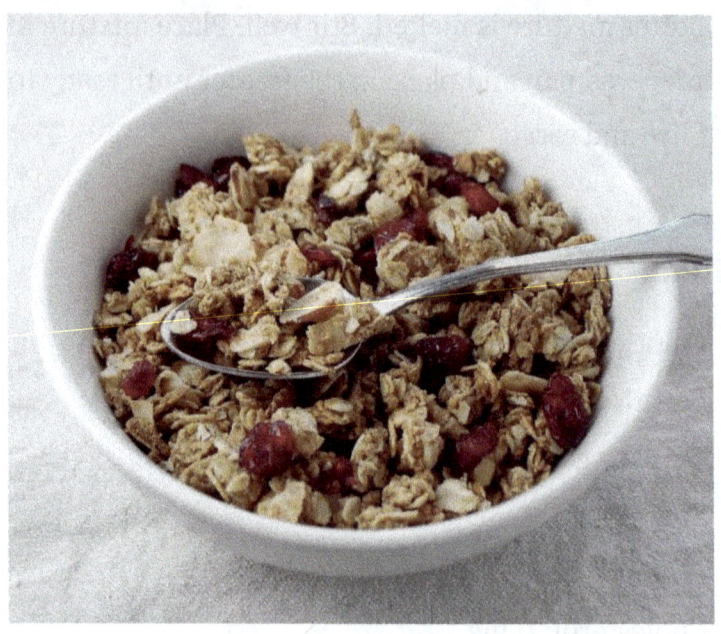

Preparation Time: 5 minutes

Cooking Time: 8 minutes

Servings: 3

Ingredients:

- 1 package of Medifast or Lean Oatmeal
- 1 packet of stevia
- 1 teaspoon of vanilla extract

- 1/2 teaspoon of apple spice or pumpkin pie spice

Directions:

1. Preheat the oven to 400° F. In a bowl, mix all the ingredients and add enough water to make the granola stay together.
2. Drop the granola onto a baking pan lined with parchment paper.
3. Bake for 8 minutes, but make sure to give the granola a good shake halfway into the cooking time for even browning.

Nutrition:

- Calories per serving: 209
- Protein: 5.8 g
- Carbohydrates: 42 g
- Fat: 3.2 g
- Sugar: 6.2 g

www.ingramcontent.com/pod-product-compliance
Lightning Source LLC
Chambersburg PA
CBHW071108030426
42336CB00013BA/1993